The Definitive Cooking Guide to Diabetic Diet Meals

Quick and Easy Recipes to Make Delicious Meals and Enjoy Your Diet

Maisie Brooks

Table of contents

Curried Carrot Soup

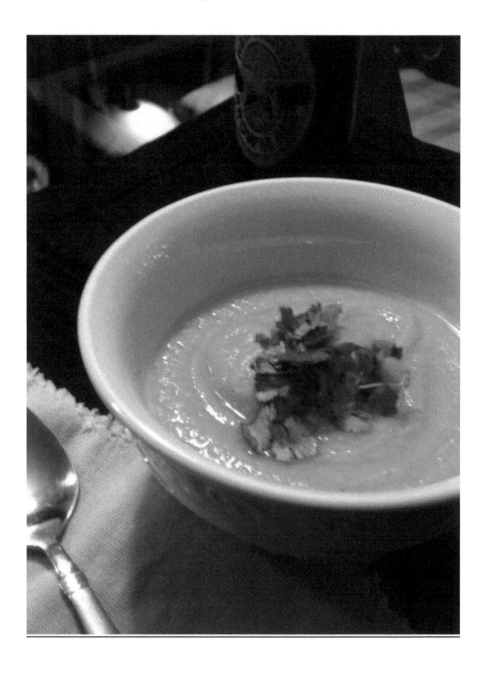

Preparation Time : 10 minutes

Cooking Time : 5 minutes

Serving : 6

Ingredients :

- 1 tablespoon extra-virgin olive oil
- 1 small onion
- 2 celery stalks
- 1½ teaspoons curry powder
- 1 teaspoon ground cumin
- 1 teaspoon minced fresh ginger
- 6 medium carrots
- 4 cups low-sodium vegetable broth
- ¼ teaspoon salt
- 1 cup canned coconut milk
- ¼ teaspoon freshly ground black pepper
- 1 tablespoon chopped fresh cilantro

Directions :

1. Heat an Pressure Pot to high and add the olive oil.

2. Sauté the onion and celery for 2 to 3 minutes. Add the curry powder, cumin, and ginger to the pot and cook until fragrant, about 30 seconds.

3. Add the carrots, vegetable broth, and salt to the pot. Close and seal, and set for 5 minutes on high. Allow the pressure to release naturally.

4. In a blender jar, carefully purée the soup in batches and transfer back to the pot.

5. Stir in the coconut milk and pepper, and heat through. Top with the cilantro and serve.

Nutrition : 145 Calories; 13g Carbohydrates; 4g Sugars

Thai Peanut, Carrot, and Shrimp Soup

Preparation Time : 10 minutes

Cooking Time : 10 minutes

Serving : 4

Ingredients :

- 1 tablespoon coconut oil
- 1 tablespoon Thai red curry paste
- ½ onion
- 3 garlic cloves
- 2 cups chopped carrots
- ½ cup whole unsalted peanuts
- 4 cups low-sodium vegetable broth
- ½ cup unsweetened plain almond milk
- ½ pound shrimp,
- Minced fresh cilantro, for garnish

Directions :

1. In a big pan, heat up oil over medium-high heat until shimmering.

2. Cook curry paste, stirring continuously, for 1 minute. Add the onion, garlic, carrots, and peanuts to the pan, and continue to cook for 2 to 3 minutes.

3. Boil broth. Reduce the heat to low and simmer for 5 to 6 minutes.

4. Purée the soup until smooth and return it to the pot. Over low heat, pour almond milk and stir to combine. Cook shrimp in the pot for 2 to 3 minutes.

5. Garnish with cilantro and serve.

Nutrition : 237 Calories; 17g Carbohydrates; 6g Sugars

Chicken Tortilla Soup

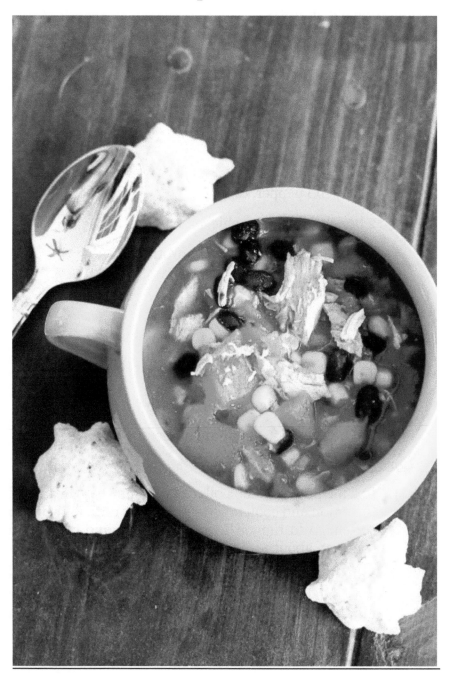

Preparation Time : 10 minutes

Cooking Time : 35 minutes

Serving : 4

Ingredients :

- 1 tablespoon extra-virgin olive oil
- 1 onion, thinly sliced
- 1 garlic clove, minced
- 1 jalapeño pepper, diced
- 2 boneless, skinless chicken breasts
- 4 cups low-sodium chicken broth
- 1 roma tomato, diced
- ½ teaspoon salt
- 2 (6-inch) corn tortillas
- Juice of 1 lime
- Minced fresh cilantro, for garnish
- ¼ cup shredded cheddar cheese, for garnish

Directions :

1. In a medium pot, cook oil over medium-high heat. Add the onion and cook for 3 to 5 minutes until it begins to soften. Add the garlic and jalapeño, and cook until fragrant, about 1 minute more.

2. Add the chicken, chicken broth, tomato, and salt to the pot and boil. Lower heat to medium and simmer mildly for 20 to 25 minutes. Remove the chicken from the pot and set aside.

3. Preheat a broiler to high.

4. Spray the tortilla strips with nonstick cooking spray and toss to coat. Spread in a single layer on a baking sheet and broil for 3 to 5 minutes, flipping once, until crisp.

5. Once chicken is cooked, shred it with two forks and return to the pot.

6. Season the soup with the lime juice. Serve hot, garnished with cilantro, cheese, and tortilla strips.

Nutrition : 191 Calories; 13g Carbohydrates; 2g Sugars

Beef and Mushroom Barley Soup

Preparation Time : 10 minutes

Cooking Time : 80 minutes

Serving : 6

Ingredients :

- 1-pound beef stew meat, cubed
- ¼ teaspoon salt
- ¼ teaspoon freshly ground black pepper
- 1 tablespoon extra-virgin olive oil
- 8 ounces sliced mushrooms
- 1 onion, chopped
- 2 carrots, chopped
- 3 celery stalks, chopped
- 6 garlic cloves, minced
- ½ teaspoon dried thyme
- 4 cups low-sodium beef broth
- 1 cup water
- ½ cup pearl barley

Directions :

1. Season the meat well.
2. In an Pressure Pot, heat the oil over high heat. Cook meat on all sides. Remove from the pot and set aside.
3. Add the mushrooms to the pot and cook for 1 to 2 minutes. Remove the mushrooms and set aside with the meat.

4. Sauté onion, carrots, and celery for 3 to 4 minutes. Add the garlic and continue to cook until fragrant, about 30 seconds longer.

5. Return the meat and mushrooms to the pot, then add the thyme, beef broth, and water. Adjust the pressure on high and cook for 15 minutes. Let the pressure release naturally.

6. Open the Pressure Pot and add the barley. Use the slow cooker function on the Pressure Pot, affix the lid (vent open), and continue to cook for 1 hour. Serve.

Nutrition : 245 Calories; 19g Carbohydrates; 3g Sugars

Cucumber, Tomato, and Avocado Salad

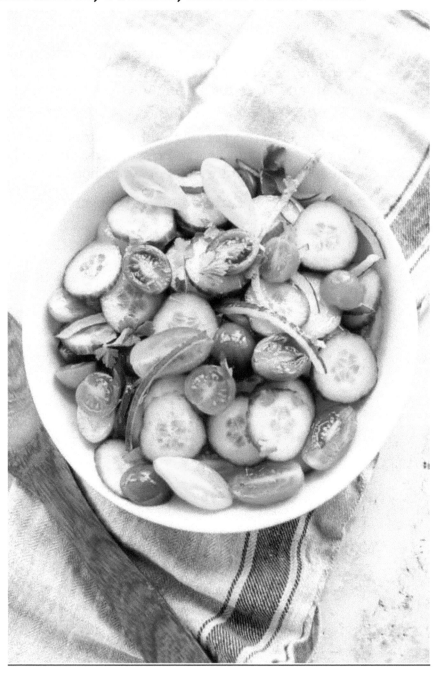

Preparation Time : 10 minutes

Cooking Time : 0 minute

Serving : 4

Ingredients :

- 1 cup cherry tomatoes
- 1 large cucumber
- 1 small red onion
- 1 avocado
- 2 tablespoons chopped fresh dill
- 2 tablespoons extra-virgin olive oil
- Juice of 1 lemon
- ¼ teaspoon salt
- ¼ teaspoon freshly ground black pepper

Directions :

1. In a big mixing bowl, mix the tomatoes, cucumber, onion, avocado, and dill.
2. In a small bowl, combine the oil, lemon juice, salt, and pepper, and mix well.
3. Drizzle the dressing over the vegetables and toss to combine. Serve.

Nutrition : 151 Calories; 11g Carbohydrates; 4g Sugars

Cabbage Slaw Salad

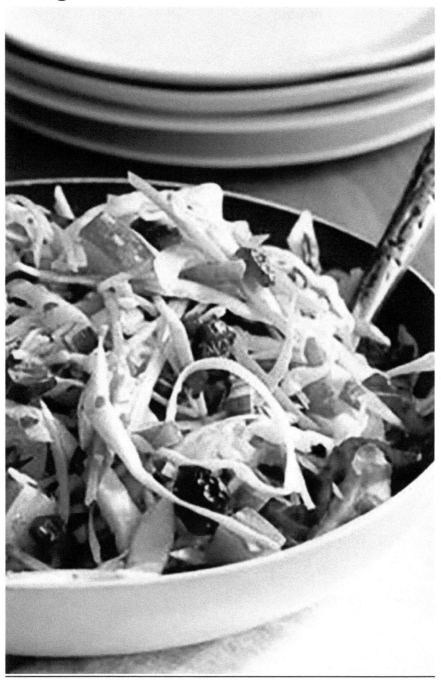

Preparation Time : 15 minutes

Cooking Time : 0 minute

Serving : 4

Ingredients :

- 2 cups green cabbage
- 2 cups red cabbage
- 2 cups grated carrots
- 3 scallions
- 2 tablespoons extra-virgin olive oil
- 2 tablespoons rice vinegar
- 1 teaspoon honey
- 1 garlic clove
- ¼ teaspoon salt

Directions :

1. Throw together the green and red cabbage, carrots, and scallions.

2. In a small bowl, whisk together the oil, vinegar, honey, garlic, and salt.

3. Pour the dressing over the veggies and mix to combine thoroughly.

4. Serve immediately, or cover and chill for several hours before serving.

Nutrition : 80 Calories; 10g Carbohydrates; 6g Sugars

Green Salad with Blackberries, Goat Cheese, and Sweet Potatoes

Preparation Time : 15 minutes

Cooking Time : 20 minutes

Serving : 4

Ingredients:

For the vinaigrette

- 1-pint blackberries
- 2 tablespoons red wine vinegar
- 1 tablespoon honey
- 3 tablespoons extra-virgin olive oil
- ¼ teaspoon salt
- Freshly ground black pepper

For the salad

- 1 sweet potato, cubed
- 1 teaspoon extra-virgin olive oil
- 8 cups salad greens (baby spinach, spicy greens, romaine)
- ½ red onion, sliced
- ¼ cup crumbled goat cheese

Directions:

For vinaigrette

1. In a blender jar, combine the blackberries, vinegar, honey, oil, salt, and pepper, and process until smooth. Set aside.

For salad

2. Preheat the oven to 425°F. Line a baking sheet with parchment paper.

3. Mix the sweet potato with the olive oil. Transfer to the prepared baking sheet and roast for 20 minutes, stirring once halfway through, until tender. Remove and cool for a few minutes.

4. In a large bowl, toss the greens with the red onion and cooled sweet potato, and drizzle with the vinaigrette. Serve topped with 1 tablespoon of goat cheese per serving.

Nutrition : 196 Calories; 21g Carbohydrates; 10g Sugars

Three Bean and Basil Salad

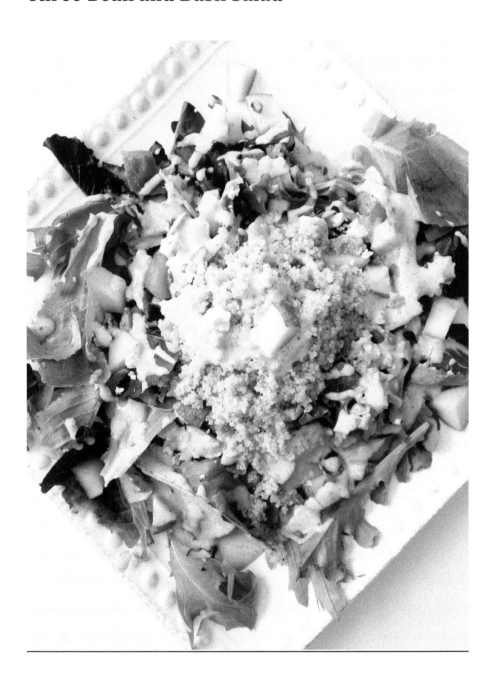

Preparation Time : 10 minutes

Cooking Time : 0 minute

Serving : 8

Ingredients :

- 1 (15-ounce) can low-sodium chickpeas
- 1 (15-ounce) can low-sodium kidney beans
- 1 (15-ounce) can low-sodium white beans
- 1 red bell pepper
- ¼ cup chopped scallions
- ¼ cup finely chopped fresh basil
- 3 garlic cloves, minced
- 2 tablespoons extra-virgin olive oil
- 1 tablespoon red wine vinegar
- 1 teaspoon Dijon mustard
- ¼ teaspoon freshly ground black pepper

Directions :

1. Toss chickpeas, kidney beans, white beans, bell pepper, scallions, basil, and garlic gently.
2. Blend together olive oil, vinegar, mustard, and pepper. Toss with the salad.
3. Wrap and chill for 1 hour.

Nutrition : 193 Calories; 29g Carbohydrates; 3g Sugars

Rainbow Black Bean Salad

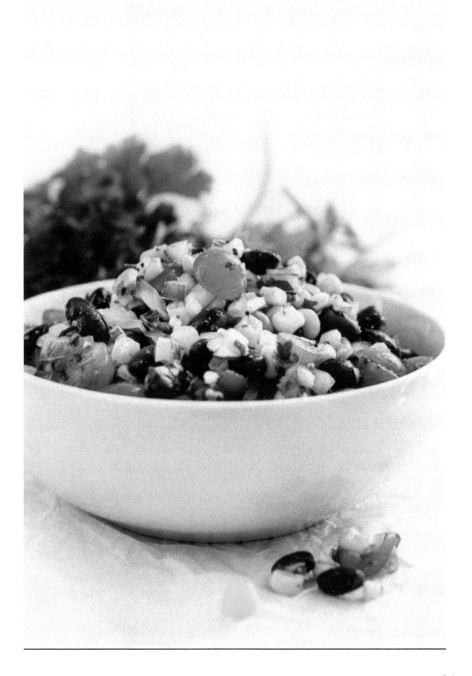

Preparation Time : 15 minutes

Cooking Time : 0 minute

Serving : 5

Ingredients :

- 1 (15-ounce) can low-sodium black beans
- 1 avocado, diced
- 1 cup cherry
- tomatoes, halved
- 1 cup chopped baby spinach
- ½ cup red bell pepper
- ¼ cup jicama
- ½ cup scallions
- ¼ cup fresh cilantro
- 2 tablespoons lime juice
- 1 tablespoon extra-virgin olive oil
- 2 garlic cloves, minced
- 1 teaspoon honey
- ¼ teaspoon salt
- ¼ teaspoon freshly ground black pepper

Directions :

1. Mix black beans, avocado, tomatoes, spinach, bell pepper, jicama, scallions, and cilantro.
2. Blend lime juice, oil, garlic, honey, salt, and pepper. Add to the salad and toss.

3. Chill for 1 hour before serving.

Nutrition : 169 Calories; 22g Carbohydrates; 3g Sugars

Warm Barley and Squash Salad

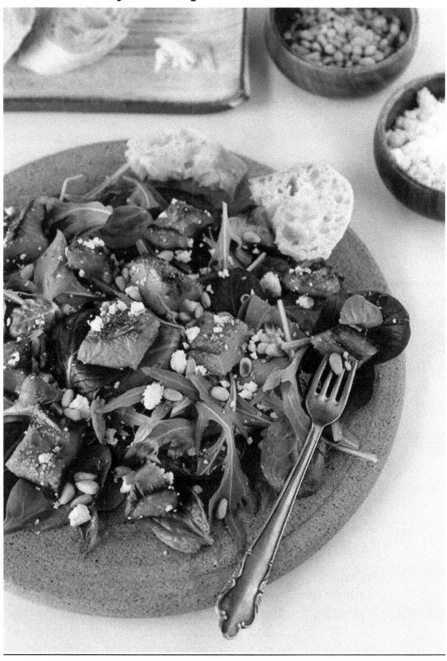

Preparation Time : 20 minutes

Cooking Time : 40 minutes

Serving : 8

Ingredients :

- 1 small butternut squash
- 3 tablespoons extra-virgin olive oil
- 2 cups broccoli florets
- 1 cup pearl barley
- 1 cup toasted chopped walnuts
- 2 cups baby kale
- ½ red onion, sliced
- 2 tablespoons balsamic vinegar
- 2 garlic cloves, minced
- ½ teaspoon salt
- ¼ teaspoon black pepper

Directions :

1. Preheat the oven to 400°F. Line a baking sheet with parchment paper.

2. Peel off the squash, and slice into dice. In a large bowl, toss the squash with 2 teaspoons of olive oil. Transfer to the prepared baking sheet and roast for 20 minutes.

3. While the squash is roasting, toss the broccoli in the same bowl with 1 teaspoon of olive oil. After 20 minutes, flip the squash and push it to one side of the baking sheet. Add the broccoli to the other side and continue to roast for 20 more minutes until tender.

4. While the veggies are roasting, in a medium pot, cover the barley with several inches of water. Boil, then adjust heat, cover, and simmer for 30 minutes until tender. Drain and rinse.

5. Transfer the barley to a large bowl, and toss with the cooked squash and broccoli, walnuts, kale, and onion.

6. In a small bowl, mix the remaining 2 tablespoons of olive oil, balsamic vinegar, garlic, salt, and pepper. Drizzle dressing over the salad and toss.

Nutrition : 274 Calories; 32g Carbohydrates; 3g Sugars

Winter Chicken and Citrus Salad

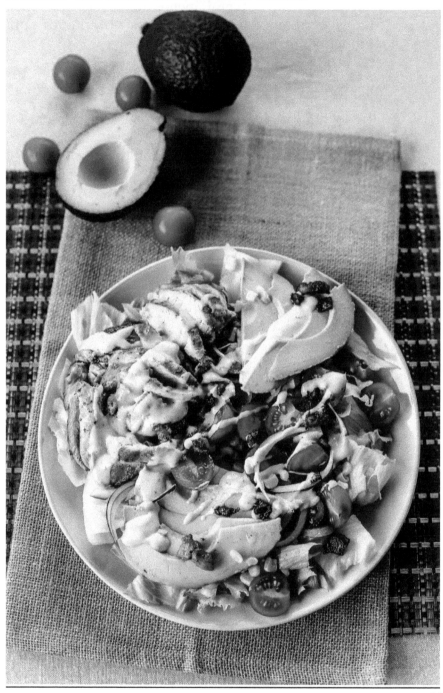

Preparation Time : 10 minutes

Cooking Time : 0 minute

Serving : 4

Ingredients :

- 4 cups baby spinach
- 2 tablespoons extra-virgin olive oil
- 1 tablespoon lemon juice
- 1/8 teaspoon salt
- 2 cups chopped cooked chicken
- 2 mandarin oranges
- ½ peeled grapefruit, sectioned
- ¼ cup sliced almonds

Directions :

1. Toss spinach with the olive oil, lemon juice, salt, and pepper.
2. Add the chicken, oranges, grapefruit, and almonds to the bowl. Toss gently.
3. Arrange on 4 plates and serve.

Nutrition : 249 Calories; 11g Carbohydrates; 7g Sugars

Pork Chops with Grape Sauce

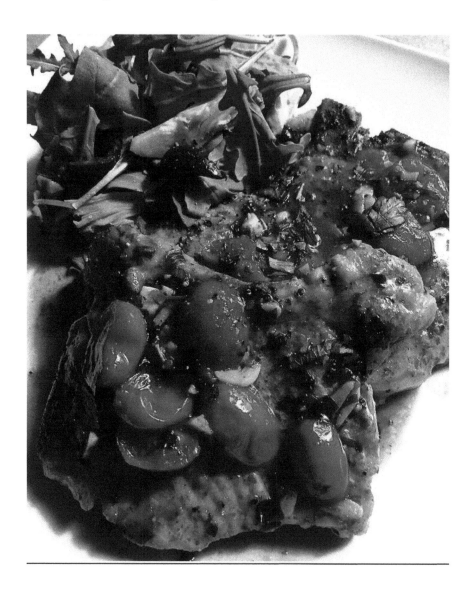

Preparation Time : 15 minutes

Cooking Time : 25 minutes

Servings : 4

Ingredients :

- Cooking spray
- 4 pork chops
- ¼ cup onion, sliced
- 1 clove garlic, minced
- 1/2 cup low-sodium chicken broth
- ¾ cup apple juice
- 1 tablespoon cornstarch
- 1 tablespoon balsamic vinegar
- 1 teaspoon honey
- 1 cup seedless red grapes, sliced in half

Directions :

1. Spray oil on your pan.
2. Put it over medium heat.
3. Add the pork chops to the pan.
4. Cook for 5 minutes per side.
5. Remove and set aside.
6. Add onion and garlic.
7. Cook for 2 minutes.
8. Pour in the broth and apple juice.
9. Bring to a boil.

10. Reduce heat to simmer.

11. Put the pork chops back to the skillet.

12. Simmer for 4 minutes.

13. In a bowl, mix the cornstarch, vinegar and honey.

14. Add to the pan.

15. Cook until the sauce has thickened.

16. Add the grapes.

17. Pour sauce over the pork chops before serving.

Nutrition : Calories 188; Total Fat 4 g; Saturated Fat 1 g; Cholesterol 47 mg; Sodium 117 mg; Total Carbohydrate 18 g; Dietary Fiber 1 g; Total Sugars 13 g; Protein19 g;Potassium 759 mg

Roasted Pork & Apples

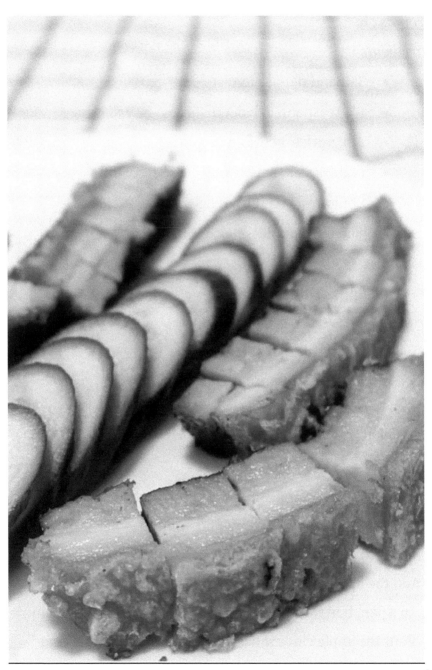

Preparation Time : 15 minutes

Cooking Time : 30 minutes

Servings : 4

Ingredients :

- Salt and pepper to taste
- 1/2 teaspoon dried, crushed
- 1 lb. pork tenderloin
- 1 tablespoon canola oil
- 1 onion, sliced into wedges
- 3 cooking apples, sliced into wedges
- 2/3 cup apple cider
- Sprigs fresh sage

Directions :

1. In a bowl, mix salt, pepper and sage.
2. Season both sides of pork with this mixture.
3. Place a pan over medium heat.
4. Brown both sides.
5. Transfer to a roasting pan.
6. Add the onion on top and around the pork.
7. Drizzle oil on top of the pork and apples.
8. Roast in the oven at 425 degrees F for 10 minutes.
9. Add the apples, roast for another 15 minutes.
10. In a pan, boil the apple cider and then simmer for 10 minutes.
11. Pour the apple cider sauce over the pork before serving.

Nutrition : Calories 239; Total Fat 6 g; Saturated Fat 1 g; Cholesterol 74 mg; Sodium 209 mg; Total Carbohydrate 22 g; Dietary Fiber 3 g;Total Sugars 16 g;Protein 24 g Potassium 655 mg

Pork with Cranberry Relish

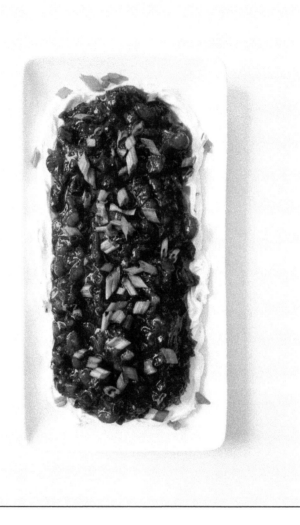

Preparation Time : 30 minutes

Cooking Time : 30 minutes

Servings : 4

Ingredients :

- 12 oz. pork tenderloin, fat trimmed and sliced crosswise
- Salt and pepper to taste
- ¼ cup all-purpose flour
- 2 tablespoons olive oil
- 1 onion, sliced thinly
- ¼ cup dried cranberries
- ¼ cup low-sodium chicken broth
- 1 tablespoon balsamic vinegar

Directions:

1. Flatten each slice of pork using a mallet.
2. In a dish, mix the salt, pepper and flour.
3. Dip each pork slice into the flour mixture.
4. Add oil to a pan over medium high heat.
5. Cook pork for 3 minutes per side or until golden crispy.
6. Transfer to a serving plate and cover with foil.
7. Cook the onion in the pan for 4 minutes.
8. Stir in the rest of the ingredients.
9. Simmer until the sauce has thickened.

Nutrition : Calories 211; Total Fat 9 g; Saturated Fat 2 g; Cholesterol 53 mg; Sodium 116 mg; Total Carbohydrate 15 g; Dietary Fiber 1 g; Total Sugars 6 g; Protein 18 g; Potassium 378 mg

Sesame Pork with Mustard Sauce

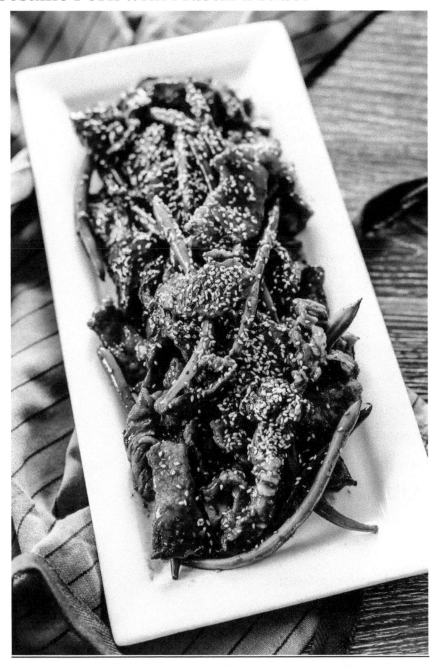

Preparation Time : 25 minutes

Cooking Time : 25 minutes

Servings : 4

Ingredients :

- 2 tablespoons low-sodium teriyaki sauce
- ¼ cup chili sauce
- 2 cloves garlic, minced
- 2 teaspoons ginger, grated
- 2 pork tenderloins
- 2 teaspoons sesame seeds
- ¼ cup low fat sour cream
- 1 teaspoon Dijon mustard
- Salt to taste
- 1 scallion, chopped

Directions :

1. Preheat your oven to 425 degrees F.
2. Mix the teriyaki sauce, chili sauce, garlic and ginger.
3. Put the pork on a roasting pan.
4. Brush the sauce on both sides of the pork.
5. Bake in the oven for 15 minutes.
6. Brush with more sauce.
7. Top with sesame seeds.
8. Roast for 10 more minutes.
9. Mix the rest of the ingredients.

10. Serve the pork with mustard sauce.

Nutrition : Calories 135; Total Fat 3 g; Saturated Fat 1 g; Cholesterol 56 mg; Sodium 302 mg; Total Carbohydrate 7 g; Dietary Fiber 1 g; Total Sugars 15 g; Protein 20 g; Potassium 755 mg

Steak with Mushroom Sauce

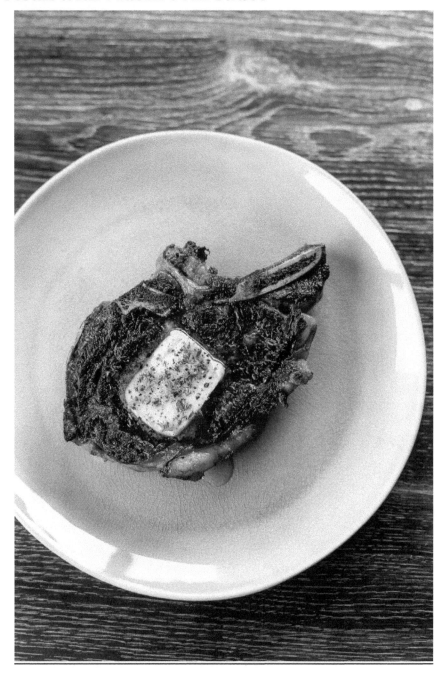

Preparation Time : 20 minutes

Cooking Time : 5 minutes

Servings : 4

Ingredients :

- 12 oz. sirloin steak, sliced and trimmed
- 2 teaspoons grilling seasoning
- 2 teaspoons oil
- 6 oz. broccoli, trimmed
- 2 cups frozen peas
- 3 cups fresh mushrooms, sliced
- 1 cup beef broth (unsalted)
- 1 tablespoon mustard
- 2 teaspoons cornstarch
- Salt to taste

Directions :

1. Preheat your oven to 350 degrees F.

2. Season meat with grilling seasoning.

3. In a pan over medium high heat, cook the meat and broccoli for 4 minutes.

4. Sprinkle the peas around the steak.

5. Put the pan inside the oven and bake for 8 minutes.

6. Remove both meat and vegetables from the pan.

7. Add the mushrooms to the pan.

8. Cook for 3 minutes.

9. Mix the broth, mustard, salt and cornstarch.

10. Add to the mushrooms.

11. Cook for 1 minute.

12. Pour sauce over meat and vegetables before serving.

Nutrition : Calories 226; Total Fat 6 g; Saturated Fat 2 g; Cholesterol 51 mg; Sodium 356 mg; Total Carbohydrate 16 g; Dietary Fiber 5 g; Total Sugars 6 g; Protein 26 g; Potassium 780 mg

Steak with Tomato & Herbs

Preparation Time : 30 minutes

Cooking Time : 30 minutes

Servings : 2

Ingredients :

- 8 oz. beef loin steak, sliced in half
- Salt and pepper to taste
- Cooking spray
- 1 teaspoon fresh basil, snipped
- ¼ cup green onion, sliced
- 1/2 cup tomato, chopped

Directions :

1. Season the steak with salt and pepper.
2. Spray oil on your pan.
3. Put the pan over medium high heat.
4. Once hot, add the steaks.
5. Reduce heat to medium.
6. Cook for 10 to 13 minutes for medium, turning once.
7. Add the basil and green onion.
8. Cook for 2 minutes.
9. Add the tomato.
10. Cook for 1 minute.
11. Let cool a little before slicing.

Nutrition : Calories 170; Total Fat 6 g; Saturated Fat 2 g;Cholesterol 66 mg;Sodium 207 mg; Total Carbohydrate 3 g;Dietary Fiber 1 g;Total Sugars 5 g ;Protein 25 g;Potassium 477 mg

Barbecue Beef Brisket

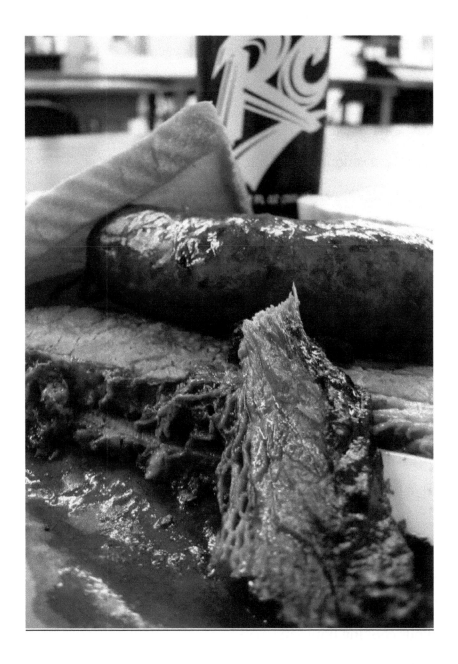

Preparation Time : 25 minutes

Cooking Time: 10 hours

Servings : 10

Ingredients :

- 4 lb. beef brisket (boneless), trimmed and sliced
- 1 bay leaf
- 2 onions, sliced into rings
- 1/2 teaspoon dried thyme, crushed
- ¼ cup chili sauce
- 1 clove garlic, minced
- Salt and pepper to taste
- 2 tablespoons light brown sugar
- 2 tablespoons cornstarch
- 2 tablespoons cold water

Directions :

1. Put the meat in a slow cooker.
2. Add the bay leaf and onion.
3. In a bowl, mix the thyme, chili sauce, salt, pepper and sugar.
4. Pour the sauce over the meat.
5. Mix well.
6. Seal the pot and cook on low heat for 10 hours.
7. Discard the bay leaf.
8. Pour cooking liquid in a pan.
9. Add the mixed water and cornstarch.

10. Simmer until the sauce has thickened.

11. Pour the sauce over the meat.

Nutrition : Calories 182; Total Fat 6 g;Saturated Fat 2 g; Cholesterol 57 mg; Sodium 217 mg; Total Sugars 4 g; Protein 20 g; Potassium 383 mg

Beef & Asparagus

Preparation Time : 15 minutes

Cooking Time : 10 minutes

Servings : 4

Ingredients :

- 2 teaspoons olive oil
- 1 lb. lean beef sirloin, trimmed and sliced
- 1 carrot, shredded
- Salt and pepper to taste
- 12 oz. asparagus, trimmed and sliced
- 1 teaspoon dried herbes de Provence, crushed
- 1/2 cup Marsala
- ¼ teaspoon lemon zest

Directions :

1. Pour oil in a pan over medium heat.
2. Add the beef and carrot.
3. Season with salt and pepper.
4. Cook for 3 minutes.
5. Add the asparagus and herbs.
6. Cook for 2 minutes.
7. Add the Marsala and lemon zest.
8. Cook for 5 minutes, stirring frequently.

Nutrition : Calories 327; Total Fat 7 g; Saturated Fat 2 g; Cholesterol 69 mg; Sodium 209 mg ;Total Carbohydrate 29 g;

Dietary Fiber 2 g; Total Sugars 3 g; Protein 28 g; Potassium 576 mg

Italian Beef

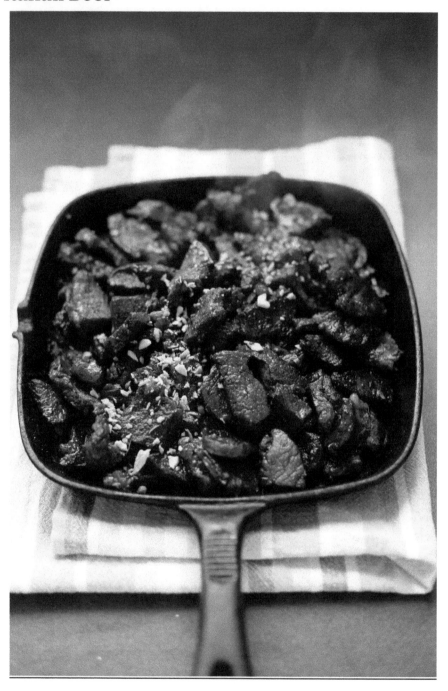

Preparation Time : 20 minutes

Cooking Time : 1 hour and 20 minutes

Servings : 4

Ingredients :

- Cooking spray
- 1 lb. beef round steak, trimmed and sliced
- 1 cup onion, chopped
- 2 cloves garlic, minced
- 1 cup green bell pepper, chopped
- 1/2 cup celery, chopped
- 2 cups mushrooms, sliced
- 14 1/2 oz. canned diced tomatoes
- 1/2 teaspoon dried basil
- ¼ teaspoon dried oregano
- 1/8 teaspoon crushed red pepper
- 2 tablespoons Parmesan cheese, grated

Directions :

1. Spray oil on the pan over medium heat.

2. Cook the meat until brown on both sides.

3. Transfer meat to a plate.

4. Add the onion, garlic, bell pepper, celery and mushroom to the pan.

5. Cook until tender.

6. Add the tomatoes, herbs, and pepper.

7. Put the meat back to the pan.

8. Simmer while covered for 1 hour and 15 minutes.

9. Stir occasionally.

10. Sprinkle Parmesan cheese on top of the dish before serving.

Nutrition : Calories 212; Total Fat 4 g; Saturated Fat 1 g; Cholesterol 51 mg; Sodium 296 mg; Total Sugars 6 g; Protein 30 g; Potassium 876 mg

Lamb with Broccoli & Carrots

Preparation Time : 20 minutes

Cooking Time : 10 minutes

Servings : 4

Ingredients :

- 2 cloves garlic, minced
- 1 tablespoon fresh ginger, grated
- ¼ teaspoon red pepper, crushed
- 2 tablespoons low-sodium soy sauce
- 1 tablespoon white vinegar
- 1 tablespoon cornstarch
- 12 oz. lamb meat, trimmed and sliced
- 2 teaspoons cooking oil
- 1 lb. broccoli, sliced into florets
- 2 carrots, sliced into strips
- ¾ cup low-sodium beef broth
- 4 green onions, chopped
- 2 cups cooked spaghetti squash pasta

Directions :

1. Combine the garlic, ginger, red pepper, soy sauce, vinegar and cornstarch in a bowl.

2. Add lamb to the marinade.

3. Marinate for 10 minutes.

4. Discard marinade.

5. In a pan over medium heat, add the oil.

6. Add the lamb and cook for 3 minutes.

7. Transfer lamb to a plate.

8. Add the broccoli and carrots.

9. Cook for 1 minute.

10. Pour in the beef broth.

11. Cook for 5 minutes.

12. Put the meat back to the pan.

13. Sprinkle with green onion and serve on top of spaghetti squash.

Nutrition: Calories 205; Total Fat 6 g; Saturated Fat 1 g; Cholesterol 40 mg; Sodium 659 mg; Total Carbohydrate 17 g

Rosemary Lamb

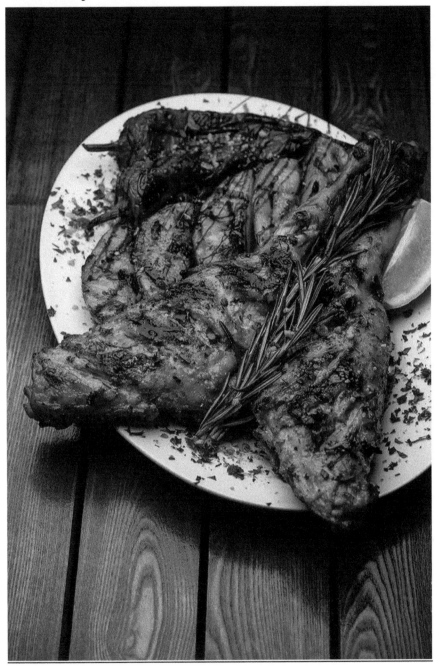

Preparation Time : 15 minutes

Cooking Time: 2 hours

Servings : 14

Ingredients:

- Salt and pepper to taste

- 2 teaspoons fresh rosemary, snipped

- 5 lb. whole leg of lamb, trimmed and cut with slits on all sides

- 3 cloves garlic, slivered

- 1 cup water

Directions :

1. Preheat your oven to 375 degrees F.

2. Mix salt, pepper and rosemary in a bowl.

3. Sprinkle mixture all over the lamb.

4. Insert slivers of garlic into the slits.

5. Put the lamb on a roasting pan.

6. Add water to the pan.

7. Roast for 2 hours.

Nutrition: Calories 136; Total Fat 4 g; Saturated Fat 1 g; Cholesterol 71 mg; Sodium 218 mg; Protein 23 g; Potassium 248 mg

Mediterranean Lamb Meatballs

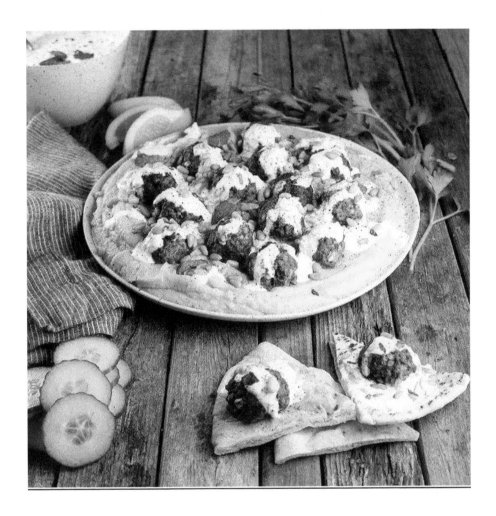

Preparation Time : 10 minutes

Cooking Time : 20 minutes

Servings: 8

Ingredients:

- 12 oz. roasted red peppers
- 1 1/2 cups whole wheat breadcrumbs
- 2 eggs, beaten
- 1/3 cup tomato sauce
- 1/2 cup fresh basil
- ¼ cup parsley, snipped
- Salt and pepper to taste
- 2 lb. lean ground lamb

Directions:

1. Preheat your oven to 350 degrees F.
2. In a bowl, mix all the ingredients and then form into meatballs.
3. Put the meatballs on a baking pan.
4. Bake in the oven for 20 minutes.

Nutrition : Calories 94; Total Fat 3 g; Saturated Fat 1 g; Cholesterol 35 mg; Sodium 170 mg; Total Carbohydrate 2 g; Dietary Fiber 1 g; Total Sugars 0 g

Blueberry and Chicken Salad

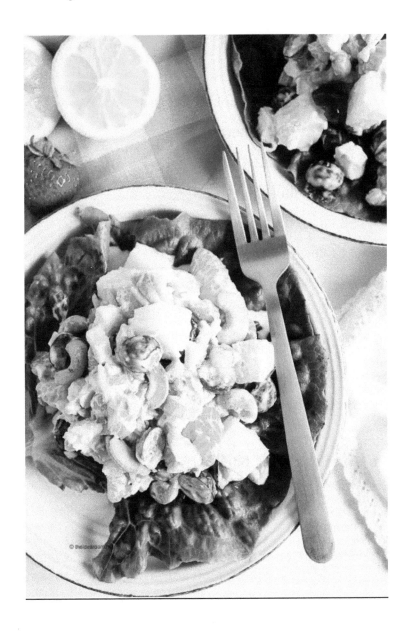

Preparation Time : 10 minutes

Cooking Time : 0 minute

Serving : 4

Ingredients :

- 2 cups chopped cooked chicken
- 1 cup fresh blueberries
- ¼ cup almonds
- 1 celery stalk
- ¼ cup red onion
- 1 tablespoon fresh basil
- 1 tablespoon fresh cilantro
- ½ cup plain, vegan mayonnaise
- ¼ teaspoon salt
- ¼ teaspoon freshly ground black pepper
- 8 cups salad greens

Directions :

1. Toss chicken, blueberries, almonds, celery, onion, basil, and cilantro.
2. Blend yogurt, salt, and pepper. Stir chicken salad to combine.
3. Situate 2 cups of salad greens on each of 4 plates and divide the chicken salad among the plates to serve.

Nutrition : 207 Calories; 11g Carbohydrates; 6g Sugars

Beef and Red Bean Chili

Preparation Time : 10 minutes

Cooking Time : 6 hours

Serving : 4

Ingredients :

- 1 cup dry red beans
- 1 tablespoon olive oil
- 2 pounds boneless beef chuck
- 1 large onion, coarsely chopped
- 1 (14 ounce) can beef broth
- 2 chipotle chili peppers in adobo sauce
- 2 teaspoons dried oregano, crushed
- 1 teaspoon ground cumin
- ½ teaspoon salt
- 1 (14.5 ounce) can tomatoes with mild green chilis
- 1 (15 ounce) can tomato sauce
- ¼ cup snipped fresh cilantro
- 1 medium red sweet pepper

Directions :

1. Rinse out the beans and place them into a Dutch oven or big saucepan, then add in water enough to cover them. Allow the beans to boil then drop the heat down. Simmer the beans without a cover for 10 minutes. Take off the heat and keep covered for an hour.

2. In a big frypan, heat up the oil upon medium-high heat, then cook onion and half the beef until they

brown a bit over medium-high heat. Move into a 3 1/2- or 4-quart crockery cooker. Do this again with what's left of the beef. Add in tomato sauce, tomatoes (not drained), salt, cumin, oregano, adobo sauce, chipotle peppers, and broth, stirring to blend. Strain out and rinse beans and stir in the cooker.

3. Cook while covered on a low setting for around 10-12 hours or on high setting for 5-6 hours. Spoon the chili into bowls or mugs and top with sweet pepper and cilantro.

Nutrition : 288 Calories; 24g Carbohydrate; 5g Sugar

Berry Apple Cider

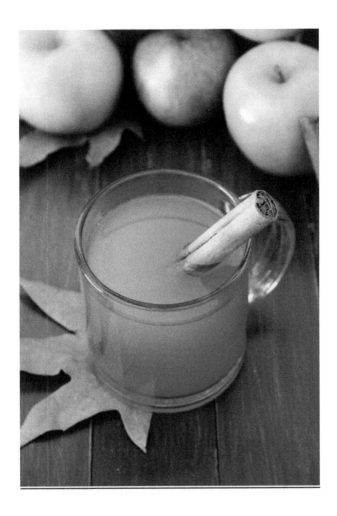

Preparation Time : 15 minutes

Cooking Time : 3 hours

Serving : 3

Ingredients :

- 4 cinnamon sticks, cut into 1-inch pieces
- 1½ teaspoons whole cloves
- 4 cups apple cider
- 4 cups low-calorie cranberry-raspberry juice drink
- 1 medium apple

Directions :

1. To make the spice bag, cut out a 6-inch square from double thick, pure cotton cheesecloth. Put in the cloves and cinnamon, then bring the corners up, tie it closed using a clean kitchen string that is pure cotton.

2. In a 3 1/2- 5-quart slow cooker, combine cranberry-raspberry juice, apple cider, and the spice bag.

3. Cook while covered over low heat setting for around 4-6 hours or on a high heat setting for 2-2 1/2 hours.

4. Throw out the spice bag. Serve right away or keep it warm while covered on warm or low-heat setting up to 2 hours, occasionally stirring. Garnish each serving with apples (thinly sliced).

Nutrition : 89 Calories; 22g Carbohydrate; 19g Sugar

Brunswick Stew

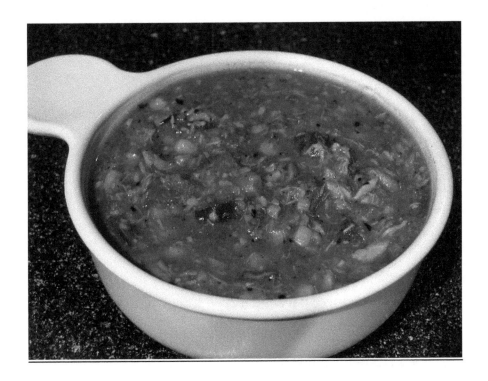

Preparation Time : 10 minutes

Cooking Time : 45 minutes

Serving : 3

Ingredients :

- 4 ounces diced salt pork
- 2 pounds chicken parts
- 8 cups water
- 3 potatoes, cubed
- 3 onions, chopped
- 1 (28 ounce) can whole peeled tomatoes
- 2 cups canned whole kernel corn
- 1 (10 ounce) package frozen lima beans
- 1 tablespoon Worcestershire sauce
- 1/2 teaspoon salt
- 1/4 teaspoon ground black pepper

Directions :

1. Mix and boil water, chicken and salt pork in a big pot on high heat. Lower heat to low. Cover then simmer until chicken is tender for 45 minutes.

2. Take out chicken. Let cool until easily handled. Take meat out. Throw out bones and skin. Chop meat to bite-sized pieces. Put back in the soup.

3. Add ground black pepper, salt, Worcestershire sauce, lima beans, corn, tomatoes, onions and potatoes. Mix well. Stir well and simmer for 1 hour, uncovered.

Nutrition : 368 Calories; 25.9g Carbohydrate; 27.9g Protein

Buffalo Chicken Salads

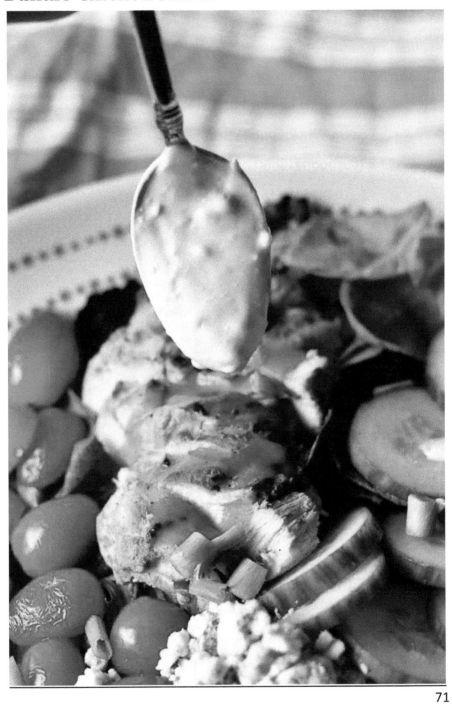

Preparation Time : 7 minutes

Cooking Time : 3 hours

Serving : 5

Ingredients :

- 1½ pounds chicken breast halves
- ½ cup Wing Time® Buffalo chicken sauce
- 4 teaspoons cider vinegar
- 1 teaspoon Worcestershire sauce
- 1 teaspoon paprika
- 1/3 cup light mayonnaise
- 2 tablespoons fat-free milk
- 2 tablespoons crumbled blue cheese
- 2 romaine hearts, chopped
- 1 cup whole grain croutons
- ½ cup very thinly sliced red onion

Directions :

1. Place chicken in a 2-quarts slow cooker. Mix together Worcestershire sauce, 2 teaspoons of vinegar and Buffalo sauce in a small bowl; pour over chicken. Dust with paprika. Close and cook for 3 hours on low-heat setting.

2. Mix the leftover 2 teaspoons of vinegar with milk and light mayonnaise together in a small bowl at serving time; mix in blue cheese. While chicken is still in the slow cooker, pull meat into bite-sized pieces using two forks.

3. Split the romaine among 6 dishes. Spoon sauce and chicken over lettuce. Pour with blue cheese dressing then add red onion slices and croutons on top.

Nutrition : 274 Calories; 11g Carbohydrate; 2g Fiber

Cacciatore Style Chicken

Preparation Time : 10 minutes

Cooking Time : 4 hours

Serving : 6

Ingredients :

- 2 cups sliced fresh mushrooms
- 1 cup sliced celery
- 1 cup chopped carrot
- 2 medium onions, cut into wedges
- 1 green, yellow, or red sweet peppers
- 4 cloves garlic, minced
- 12 chicken drumsticks
- ½ cup chicken broth
- ¼ cup dry white wine
- 2 tablespoons quick-cooking tapioca
- 2 bay leaves
- 1 teaspoon dried oregano, crushed
- 1 teaspoon sugar
- ½ teaspoon salt
- ¼ teaspoon pepper
- 1 (14.5 ounce) can diced tomatoes
- 1/3 cup tomato paste
- Hot cooked pasta or rice

<u>Directions</u> :

1. Mix garlic, sweet pepper, onions, carrot, celery and mushrooms in a 5- or 6-qt. slow cooker. Cover veggies with the chicken. Add pepper, salt, sugar, oregano, bay leaves, tapioca, wine and broth.

2. Cover. Cook for 3–3 1/2 hours on high-heat setting.

3. Take chicken out; keep warm. Discard bay leaves. Turn to high-heat setting if using low-heat setting. Mix tomato paste and undrained tomatoes in. Cover. Cook on high-heat setting for 15 more minutes. Serving: Put veggie mixture on top of pasta and chicken.

<u>Nutrition</u> : 324 Calories; 7g Sugar; 35g Carbohydrate

Carnitas Tacos

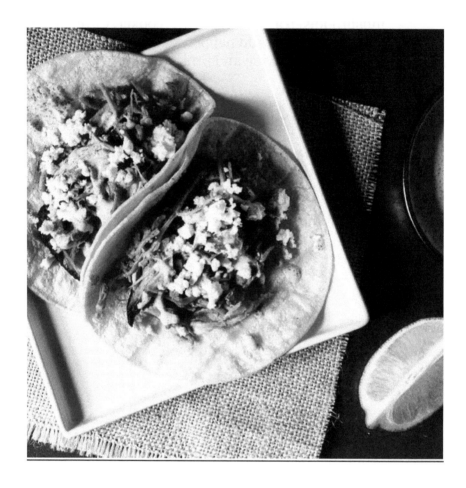

Preparation Time : 10 minutes

Cooking Time : 5 hours

Serving : 4

Ingredients :

- 3 to 3½-pound bone-in pork shoulder roast
- ½ cup chopped onion
- 1/3 cup orange juice
- 1 tablespoon ground cumin
- 1½ teaspoons kosher salt
- 1 teaspoon dried oregano, crushed
- ¼ teaspoon cayenne pepper
- 1 lime
- 2 (5.3 ounce) containers plain low-fat Greek yogurt
- 1 pinch kosher salt
- 16 (6 inch) soft yellow corn tortillas, such as Mission® brand
- 4 leaves green cabbage, quartered
- 1 cup very thinly sliced red onion
- 1 cup salsa (optional)

Directions :

1. Take off meat from the bone; throw away bone. Trim meat fat. Slice meat into 2 to 3-inch pieces; put in a slow cooker of 3 1/2 or 4-quart in size. Mix in cayenne, oregano, salt, cumin, orange juice and onion.

2. Cover and cook for 4 to 5 hours on high. Take out meat from the cooker. Shred meat with two forks. Mix in enough cooking liquid to moisten.

3. Take out 1 teaspoon zest (put aside) for lime crema, then squeeze 2 tablespoons lime juice. Mix dash salt, yogurt, and lime juice in a small bowl.

4. Serve lime crema, salsa (if wished), red onion and cabbage with meat in tortillas. Scatter with lime zest.

Nutrition : 301 Calories; 28g Carbohydrate; 7g Sugar

Chicken Chili

Preparation Time : 6 minutes

Cooking Time : 1 hour

Serving : 4

Ingredients :

- 3 tablespoons vegetable oil
- 2 cloves garlic, minced
- 1 green bell pepper, chopped
- 1 onion, chopped
- 1 stalk celery, sliced
- 1/4-pound mushrooms, chopped
- 1-pound chicken breast
- 1 tablespoon chili powder
- 1 teaspoon dried oregano
- 1 teaspoon ground cumin
- 1/2 teaspoon paprika
- 1/2 teaspoon cocoa powder
- 1/4 teaspoon salt
- 1 pinch crushed red pepper flakes
- 1 pinch ground black pepper
- 1 (14.5 oz) can tomatoes with juice
- 1 (19 oz) can kidney beans

Directions :

1. Fill 2 tablespoons of oil into a big skillet and heat it at moderate heat. Add mushrooms, celery, onion, bell pepper and garlic, sautéing for 5 minutes. Put it to one side.

2. Insert the leftover 1 tablespoon of oil into the skillet. At high heat, cook the chicken until browned and its exterior turns firm. Transfer the vegetable mixture back into skillet.

3. Stir in ground black pepper, hot pepper flakes, salt, cocoa powder, paprika, oregano, cumin and chili powder. Continue stirring for several minutes to avoid burning. Pour in the beans and tomatoes and lead the entire mixture to boiling point then adjust the setting to low heat. Place a lid on the skillet and leave it simmering for 15 minutes. Uncover the skillet and leave it simmering for another 15 minutes.

Nutrition : 308 Calories; 25.9g Carbohydrate; 29g Protein

Chicken Vera Cruz

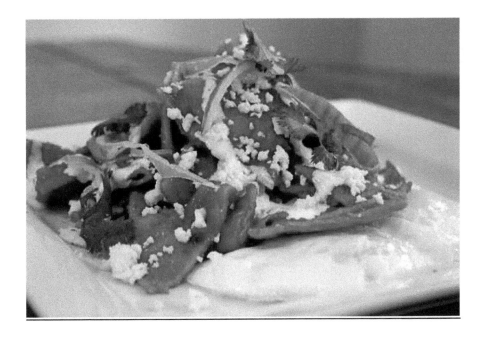

Preparation Time : 7 minutes

Cooking Time : 10 hours

Serving : 5

Ingredients :

- 1 medium onion, cut into wedges
- 1-pound yellow-skin potatoes
- 6 skinless, boneless chicken thighs
- 2 (14.5 oz.) cans no-salt-added diced tomatoes
- 1 fresh jalapeño chili pepper
- 2 tablespoons Worcestershire sauce
- 1 tablespoon chopped garlic
- 1 teaspoon dried oregano, crushed
- ¼ teaspoon ground cinnamon
- 1/8 teaspoon ground cloves
- ½ cup snipped fresh parsley
- ¼ cup chopped pimiento-stuffed green olives

Directions:

1. Put onion in a 3 1/2- or 4-quart slow cooker. Place chicken thighs and potatoes on top. Drain and discard juices from a can of tomatoes. Stir undrained and drained tomatoes, cloves, cinnamon, oregano, garlic, Worcestershire sauce and jalapeño pepper together in a bowl. Pour over all in the cooker.

2. Cook with a cover for 10 hours on low-heat setting.

3. To make the topping: Stir chopped pimiento-stuffed green olives and snipped fresh parsley together in a

small bowl. Drizzle the topping over each serving of chicken.

Nutrition : 228 Calories; 9g Sugar; 25g Carbohydrate

Chicken and Cornmeal Dumplings

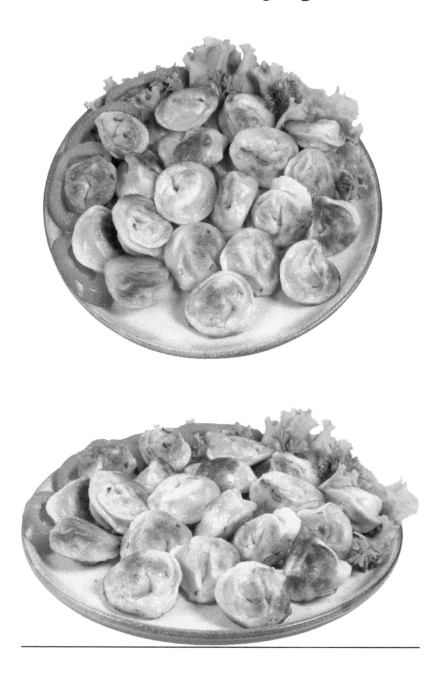

Preparation Time : 8 minutes

Cooking Time : 8 hours

Serving : 4

Ingredients:

Chicken and Vegetable Filling

- 2 medium carrots, thinly sliced
- 1 stalk celery, thinly sliced
- 1/3 cup corn kernels
- ½ of a medium onion, thinly sliced
- 2 cloves garlic, minced
- 1 teaspoon snipped fresh rosemary
- ¼ teaspoon ground black pepper
- 2 chicken thighs, skinned
- 1 cup reduced sodium chicken broth
- ½ cup fat-free milk
- 1 tablespoon all-purpose flour

Cornmeal Dumplings

- ¼ cup flour
- ¼ cup cornmeal
- ½ teaspoon baking powder
- 1 egg white
- 1 tablespoon fat-free milk
- 1 tablespoon canola oil

Directions :

1. Mix 1/4 teaspoon pepper, carrots, garlic, celery, rosemary, corn, and onion in a 1 1/2 or 2-quart slow cooker. Place chicken on top. Pour the broth atop mixture in the cooker.

2. Close and cook on low-heat for 7 to 8 hours.

3. If cooking with the low-heat setting, switch to high-heat setting (or if heat setting is not available, continue to cook). Place the chicken onto a cutting board and let to cool slightly. Once cool enough to handle, chop off chicken from bones and get rid of the bones. Chop the chicken and place back into the mixture in cooker. Mix flour and milk in a small bowl until smooth. Stir into the mixture in cooker.

4. Drop the Cornmeal Dumplings dough into 4 mounds atop hot chicken mixture using two spoons. Cover and cook for 20 to 25 minutes more or until a toothpick come out clean when inserted into a dumpling. (Avoid lifting lid when cooking.) Sprinkle each of the serving with coarse pepper if desired.

5. Mix together 1/2 teaspoon baking powder, 1/4 cup flour, a dash of salt and 1/4 cup cornmeal in a medium bowl. Mix 1 tablespoon canola oil, 1 egg white and 1 tablespoon fat-free milk in a small bowl. Pour the egg mixture into the flour mixture. Mix just until moistened.

Nutrition : 369 Calories; 9g Sugar; 47g Carbohydrate

Chicken and Pepperoni

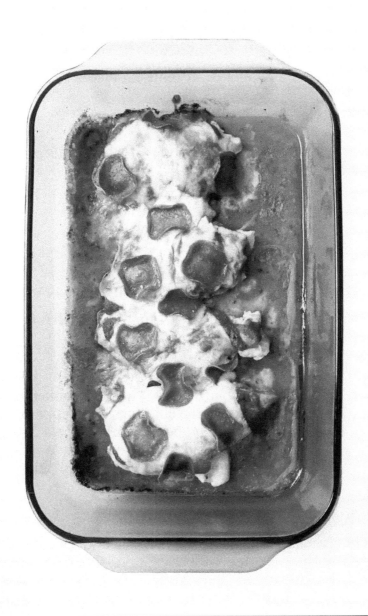

Preparation Time : 4 minutes

Cooking Time : 4 hours

Serving : 5

Ingredients :

- 3½ to 4 pounds meaty chicken pieces
- 1/8 teaspoon salt
- 1/8 teaspoon black pepper
- 2 ounces sliced turkey pepperoni
- ¼ cup sliced pitted ripe olives
- ½ cup reduced-sodium chicken broth
- 1 tablespoon tomato paste
- 1 teaspoon dried Italian seasoning, crushed
- ½ cup shredded part-skim mozzarella cheese (2 ounces)

Directions :

1. Put chicken into a 3 1/2 to 5-qt. slow cooker. Sprinkle pepper and salt on the chicken. Slice pepperoni slices in half. Put olives and pepperoni into the slow cooker. In a small bowl, blend Italian seasoning, tomato paste and chicken broth together. Transfer the mixture into the slow cooker.

2. Cook with a cover for 3-3 1/2 hours on high.

3. Transfer the olives, pepperoni and chicken onto a serving platter with a slotted spoon. Discard the cooking liquid. Sprinkle cheese over the chicken. Use foil to loosely cover and allow to sit for 5 minutes to melt the cheese.

Nutrition : 243 Calories; 1g Carbohydrate; 41g Protein

Chicken and Sausage Gumbo

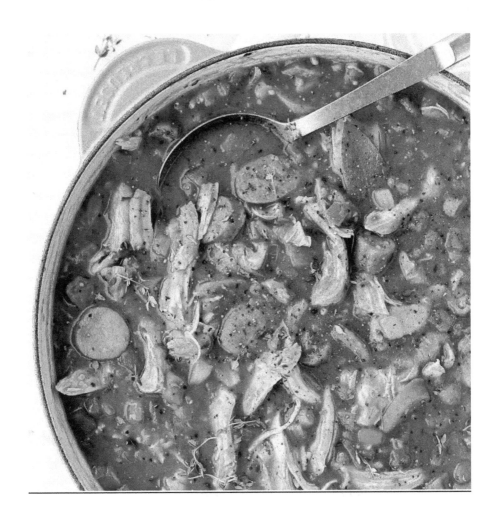

Preparation Time : 6 minutes

Cooking Time : 4 hours

Serving : 5

Ingredients :

- 1/3 cup all-purpose flour
- 1 (14 ounce) can reduced-sodium chicken broth
- 2 cups chicken breast
- 8 ounces smoked turkey sausage links
- 2 cups sliced fresh okra
- 1 cup water
- 1 cup coarsely chopped onion
- 1 cup sweet pepper
- ½ cup sliced celery
- 4 cloves garlic, minced
- 1 teaspoon dried thyme
- ½ teaspoon ground black pepper
- ¼ teaspoon cayenne pepper
- 3 cups hot cooked brown rice

Directions :

1. To make the roux: Cook the flour upon a medium heat in a heavy medium-sized saucepan, stirring periodically, for roughly 6 minutes or until the flour browns. Take off the heat and slightly cool, then slowly stir in the broth. Cook the roux until it bubbles and thickens up.

2. Pour the roux in a 3 1/2- or 4-quart slow cooker, then add in cayenne pepper, black pepper, thyme, garlic, celery, sweet pepper, onion, water, okra, sausage, and chicken.

3. Cook the soup covered on a high setting for 3 - 3 1/2 hours. Take the fat off the top and serve atop hot cooked brown rice.

Nutrition : 230 Calories; 3g Sugar; 19g Protein

Chicken, Barley, and Leek Stew

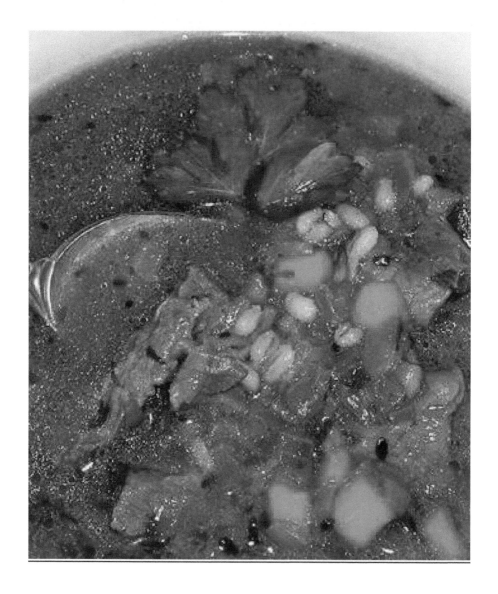

Preparation Time : 10 minutes

Cooking Time : 3 hours

Serving : 2

Ingredients :

- 1-pound chicken thighs
- 1 tablespoon olive oil
- 1 (49 ounce) can reduced-sodium chicken broth
- 1 cup regular barley (not quick-cooking)
- 2 medium leeks, halved lengthwise and sliced
- 2 medium carrots, thinly sliced
- 1½ teaspoons dried basil or Italian seasoning, crushed
- ¼ teaspoon cracked black pepper

Directions :

1. In the big skillet, cook the chicken in hot oil till becoming brown on all sides. In the 4-5-qt. slow cooker, whisk the pepper, dried basil, carrots, leeks, barley, chicken broth and chicken.

2. Keep covered and cooked over high heat setting for 2 – 2.5 hours or till the barley softens. As you wish, drizzle with the parsley or fresh basil prior to serving.

Nutrition : 248 Calories; 6g Fiber; 27g Carbohydrate

Cider Pork Stew

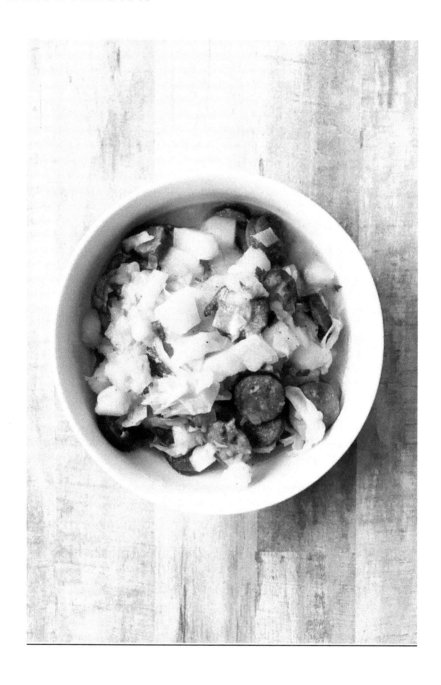

Preparation Time : 9 minutes

Cooking Time : 12 hours

Serving: 3

Ingredients :

- 2 pounds pork shoulder roast
- 3 medium cubed potatoes
- 3 medium carrots
- 2 medium onions, sliced
- 1 cup coarsely chopped apple
- ½ cup coarsely chopped celery
- 3 tablespoons quick-cooking tapioca
- 2 cups apple juice
- 1 teaspoon salt
- 1 teaspoon caraway seeds
- ¼ teaspoon black pepper

Directions :

1. Chop the meat into 1-in. cubes. In the 3.5- 5.5 qt. slow cooker, mix the tapioca, celery, apple, onions, carrots, potatoes and meat. Whisk in pepper, caraway seeds, salt and apple juice.

2. Keep covered and cook over low heat setting for 10-12 hours. If you want, use the celery leaves to decorate each of the servings.

Nutrition : 244 Calories; 5g Fiber; 33g Carbohydrate

Creamy Chicken Noodle Soup

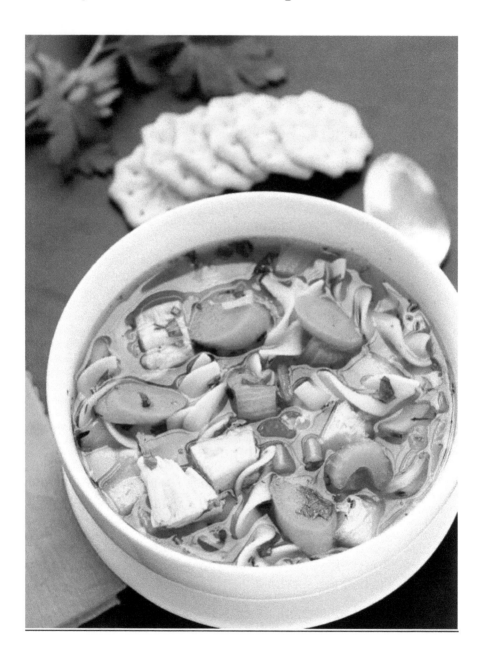

Preparation Time : 7 minutes

Cooking Time : 8 hours

Serving : 4

Ingredients :

- 1 (32 fluid ounce) container reduced-sodium chicken broth
- 3 cups water
- 2½ cups chopped cooked chicken
- 3 medium carrots, sliced
- 3 stalks celery
- 1½ cups sliced fresh mushrooms
- ¼ cup chopped onion
- 1½ teaspoons dried thyme, crushed
- ¾ teaspoon garlic-pepper seasoning
- 3 ounces reduced-fat cream cheese (Neufchâtel), cut up
- 2 cups dried egg noodles

Directions :

1. Mix together the garlic-pepper seasoning, thyme, onion, mushrooms, celery, carrots, chicken, water and broth in a 5 to 6-quart slow cooker.

2. Put cover and let it cook for 6-8 hours on low-heat setting.

3. Increase to high-heat setting if you are using low-heat setting. Mix in the cream cheese until blended. Mix in uncooked noodles. Put cover and let it cook for an

additional 20-30 minutes or just until the noodles become tender.

Nutrition : 170 Calories; 3g Sugar; 2g Fiber

Cuban Pulled Pork Sandwich

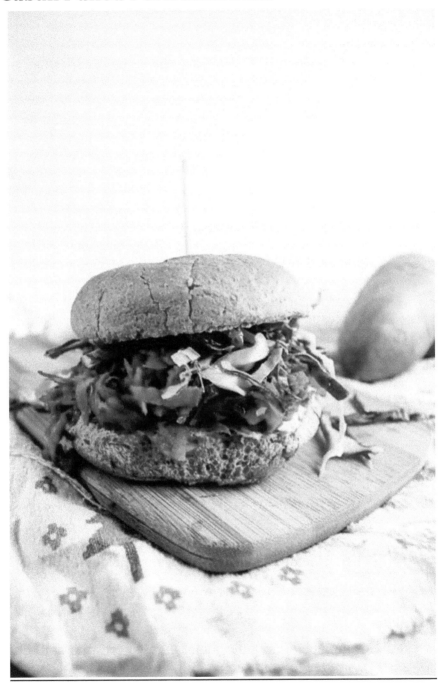

Preparation Time : 6 minutes

Cooking Time : 5 hours

Serving : 5

Ingredients :

- 1 teaspoon dried oregano, crushed
- ¾ teaspoon ground cumin
- ½ teaspoon ground coriander
- ¼ teaspoon salt
- ¼ teaspoon black pepper
- ¼ teaspoon ground allspice
- 1 2 to 2½-pound boneless pork shoulder roast
- 1 tablespoon olive oil
- Nonstick cooking spray
- 2 cups sliced onions
- 2 green sweet peppers, cut into bite-size strips
- ½ to 1 fresh jalapeño pepper
- 4 cloves garlic, minced
- ¼ cup orange juice
- ¼ cup lime juice
- 6 heart-healthy wheat hamburger buns, toasted
- 2 tablespoons jalapeño mustard

Directions :

1. Mix allspice, oregano, black pepper, cumin, salt, and coriander together in a small bowl. Press each side of

the roast into the spice mixture. On medium-high heat, heat oil in a big non-stick pan; put in roast. Cook for 5mins until both sides of the roast is light brown, turn the roast one time.

2. Using a cooking spray, grease a 3 1/2 or 4qt slow cooker; arrange the garlic, onions, jalapeno, and green peppers in a layer. Pour in lime juice and orange juice. Slice the roast if needed to fit inside the cooker; put on top of the vegetables covered or 4 1/2-5hrs on high heat setting.

3. Move roast to a cutting board using a slotted spoon. Drain the cooking liquid and keep the jalapeno, green peppers, and onions. Shred the roast with 2 forks then place it back in the cooker. Remove fat from the liquid. Mix half cup of cooking liquid and reserved vegetables into the cooker. Pour in more cooking liquid if desired. Discard the remaining cooking liquid.

4. Slather mustard on rolls. Split the meat between the bottom roll halves. Add avocado on top if desired. Place the roll tops to sandwiches.

Nutrition : 379 Calories; 32g Carbohydrate; 4g Fiber

Gazpacho

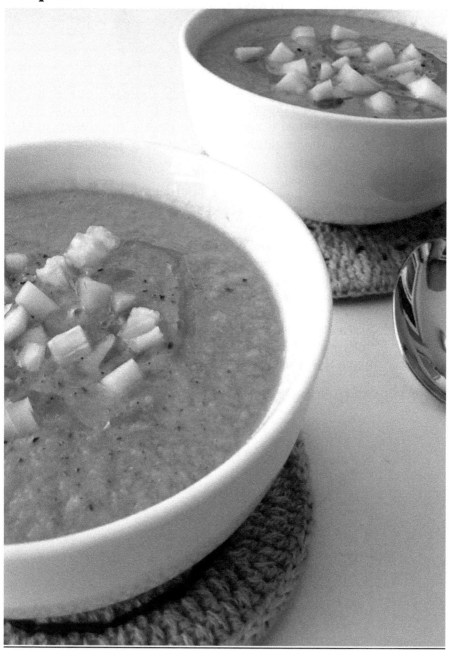

Preparation Time : 15 minutes

Cooking Time : 0 minute

Serving : 4

Ingredients :

- 3 pounds ripe tomatoes
- 1 cup low-sodium tomato juice
- ½ red onion, chopped
- 1 cucumber
- 1 red bell pepper
- 2 celery stalks
- 2 tablespoons parsley
- 2 garlic cloves
- 2 tablespoons extra-virgin olive oil
- 2 tablespoons red wine vinegar
- 1 teaspoon honey
- ½ teaspoon salt
- ¼ teaspoon freshly ground black pepper

Direction s:

1. In a blender jar, combine the tomatoes, tomato juice, onion, cucumber, bell pepper, celery, parsley, garlic, olive oil, vinegar, honey, salt, and pepper. Pulse until blended but still slightly chunky.

2. Adjust the seasonings as needed and serve.

Nutrition : 170 Calories; 24g Carbohydrates; 16g Sugars

Tomato and Kale Soup

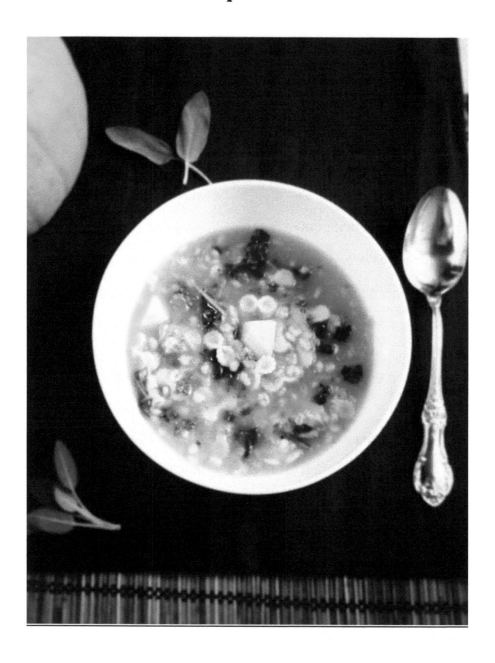

Preparation Time : 10 minutes

Cooking Time : 15 minutes

Servings: 4

Ingredients :

- 1 tablespoon extra-virgin olive oil

- 1 medium onion

- 2 carrots

- 3 garlic cloves

- 4 cups low-sodium vegetable broth

- 1 (28-ounce) can crushed tomatoes

- ½ teaspoon dried oregano

- ¼ teaspoon dried basil

- 4 cups chopped baby kale leaves

- ¼ teaspoon salt

Directions :

1. In a huge pot, heat up oil over medium heat. Sauté onion and carrots for 3 to 5 minutes. Add the garlic and sauté for 30 seconds more, until fragrant.

2. Add the vegetable broth, tomatoes, oregano, and basil to the pot and boil. Decrease the heat to low and simmer for 5 minutes.

3. Using an immersion blender, purée the soup.

4. Add the kale and simmer for 3 more minutes. Season with the salt. Serve immediately.

Nutrition: 170 Calories; 31g Carbohydrates; 13g Sugars

Comforting Summer Squash Soup with Crispy Chickpeas

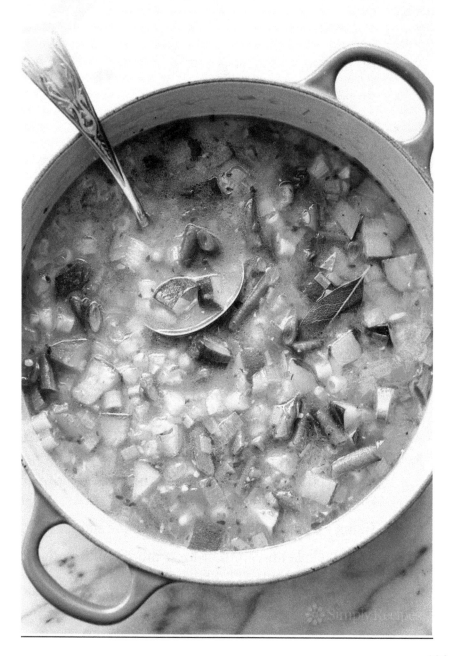

Preparation Time : 10 minutes

Cooking Time : 20 minutes

Serving : 4

Ingredients :

- 1 (15-ounce) can low-sodium chickpeas
- 1 teaspoon extra-virgin olive oil
- ¼ teaspoon smoked paprika
- Pinch salt, plus ½ teaspoon
- 3 medium zucchinis
- 3 cups low-sodium vegetable broth
- ½ onion
- 3 garlic cloves
- 2 tablespoons plain low-fat Greek yogurt
- Freshly ground black pepper

Directions :

1. Preheat the oven to 425°F. Line a baking sheet with parchment paper.

2. In a medium mixing bowl, toss the chickpeas with 1 teaspoon of olive oil, the smoked paprika, and a pinch salt. Transfer to the prepared baking sheet and roast until crispy, about 20 minutes, stirring once. Set aside.

3. Meanwhile, in a medium pot, heat the remaining 1 tablespoon of oil over medium heat.

4. Add the zucchini, broth, onion, and garlic to the pot, and boil. Simmer, and cook for 20 minutes.

5. In a blender jar, purée the soup. Return to the pot.

6. Add the yogurt, remaining ½ teaspoon of salt, and pepper, and stir well. Serve topped with the roasted chickpeas.

Nutrition : 188 Calories; 24g Carbohydrates; 7g Sugars